Keto Diet Cookbook

Quick, Easy and Affordable Recipes to Enjoy the Keto Lifestyle. Ketogenic Diet Recipes for Healthy Living, Weight Loss, Lower Cholesterol, Reverse Disease and Balance Hormones.

Alexangel Kitchen

Just for Our Readers

To Thank You for Purchasing the Book, for a limited time, you can get a Special FREE BOOK from Alexangel Kitchen

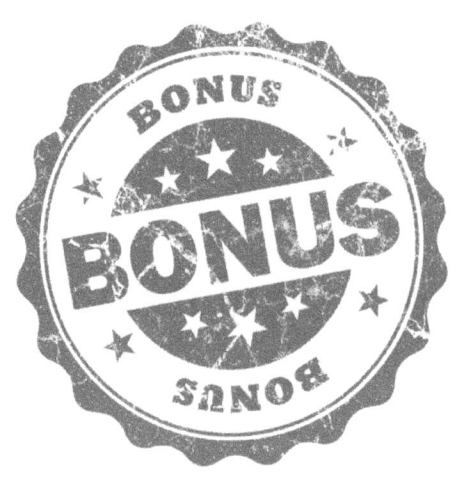

Just go to https://alexangelkitchen.com/ to download your FREE BOOK

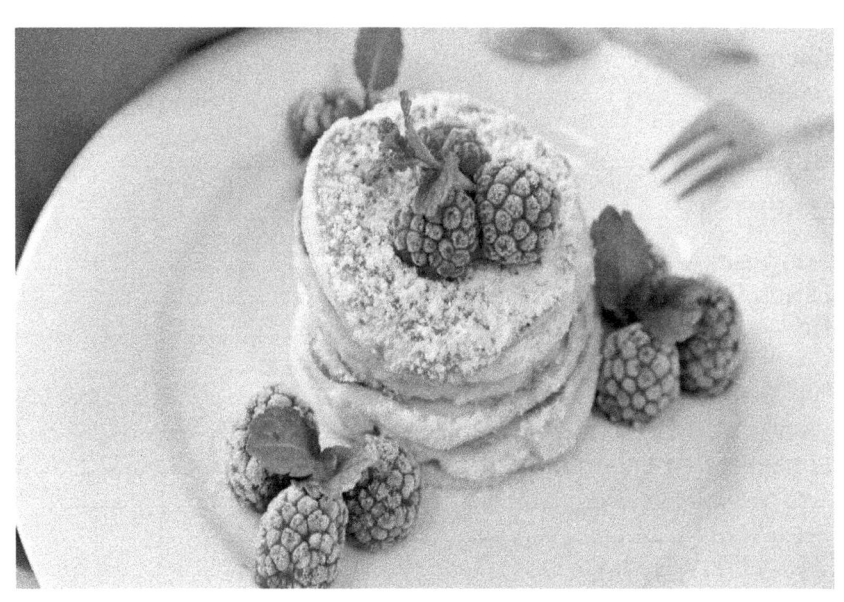

Table of Contents

- Table of Contents 4
- **INTRODUCTION** 11
  - Lemon Mushrooms 17
  - Feta Psiti 18
  - Cauliflower Queso 20
  - Sweet Smokies 22
  - Rosemary Chicken Wings 23
  - Classic Meatballs 24
  - Bacon Deviled Eggs 26
  - Spinach Dip 28
  - Sausage Balls 29
  - BLT Dip 30
- **DESSERTS** 32
  - Southern Apple Pie 32
  - Lemon Cheesecake 34
  - No-Guilt Chocolate Cake 36
  - Cheese Berry Pie 38
  - The Best Cookies 40
  - Salty Caramel Cake 42
  - Luscious Red Velvet Cake 44
  - Southern Pecan Pie 46
  - Pepperoni Pizza Cups 48
  - White Pizza Frittata 50
  - Walnut Cookies 52
  - Fathead Sausage Rolls 54
  - Chia Seed Crackers 56
  - Cheesy Biscuits 58
  - Chicken rolls with pesto 60
  - Sweet and sour sauce: 62
  - Coconut Curry Cauliflower Soup 63
  - Chocolate Cake with Vanilla Glaze 65
  - Rum Truffles 68
  - Mint Cake 70
  - Vanilla Cherry Panna Cotta 73

Keto Berry Pancakes 75
Mocha Pots de Crème 77
Lemon Cake with Berry Syrup 79
Easy Rum Cheesecake 81
Lemon Vegan Cake 83
Dark Chocolate Granola Bars 85
Blueberry Crisp 87
Chocolate Chip Quinoa Granola Bars 89
Strawberry Granita 91
Apple Fritters 93
Roasted Bananas 95
Berry-Banana Yogurt 97
Avocado Chocolate Mousse 99
Apricot Squares 100
Raw Black Forest Brownies 101
Berry Parfait 102
Sherbet Pineapple 103

SNACKS 105

Blueberry Scones 105
Homemade Graham Crackers 107

© Copyright 2020 by Alexangel Kitchen - All rights reserved.

The following Book is reproduced below with the goal of providing information that is as accurate and reliable as possible. Regardless, purchasing this Book can be seen as consent to the fact that both the publisher and the author of this book are in no way experts on the topics discussed within and that any recommendations or suggestions that are made herein are for entertainment purposes only. Professionals should be consulted as needed prior to undertaking any of the action endorsed herein.

This declaration is deemed fair and valid by both the American Bar Association and the Committee of Publishers Association and is legally binding throughout the United States.

Furthermore, the transmission, duplication, or reproduction of any of the following work including specific information will be considered an illegal act irrespective of if it is done electronically or in print. This extends to creating a secondary or tertiary copy of the work or a recorded copy and is only allowed with the express written consent from the Publisher. All additional right reserved.

The information in the following pages is broadly considered a truthful and accurate account of facts and as such, any inattention, use, or misuse of the information in question by the reader will render any resulting actions solely under their purview. There are no scenarios in which the publisher or the original author of this work can be in any fashion deemed liable for any hardship or damages that may befall them after undertaking information described herein.

Additionally, the information in the following pages is intended only for informational purposes and should thus be thought of as universal. As befitting its nature, it is presented without assurance regarding its prolonged validity or interim quality. Trademarks that are mentioned are done without written consent and can in no way be considered an endorsement from the trademark holder.

INTRODUCTION

So the Ketogenic Diet is all about reducing the amount of carbohydrates you eat. Does this mean you won't get the kind of energy you need for the day? Of course not! It only means that now, your body has to find other possible sources of energy. Do you know where they will be getting that energy?

Even before we talk about how to do keto – it's important to first consider why this particular diet works. What actually happens to your body to make you lose weight?

As you probably know, the body uses food as an energy source. Everything you eat is turned into energy, so that you can get up and do whatever you need to accomplish for the day. The main energy source is sugar so what happens is that you eat something, the body breaks it down into sugar, and the sugar is processed into energy. Typically, the "sugar" is taken directly from the food you eat so if you eat just the right amount of food, then your body is fueled for the whole day. If you eat too much, then the sugar is stored in your body – hence the accumulation of fat.

But what happens if you eat less food? This is where the Ketogenic Diet comes in. You see, the process of creating sugar from food is usually faster if the food happens to be rich in carbohydrates. Bread, rice, grain, pasta – all of these are carbohydrates and they're the easiest food types to turn into energy.

So here's the situation – you are eating less carbohydrates every day. To keep you energetic, the body breaks down the stored fat and turns them into molecules called ketone bodies. The process of turning the fat into ketone bodies is called "Ketosis" and obviously – this is where the name of the Ketogenic Diet comes from. The ketone bodies take the place of glucose in keeping you energetic. As long as you keep your carbohydrates reduced, the body will keep getting its energy from your body fat.

The Ketogenic Diet is often praised for its simplicity and when you look at it properly, the process is really straightforward. The Science behind the effectivity of the diet is also well-documented, and has been proven multiple times by different medical fields. For example, an article on Diet Review by Harvard provided a lengthy discussion on how the Ketogenic Diet works and why it is so effective for those who choose to use this diet.

But Fat Is the Enemy…Or Is It?

No – fat is NOT the enemy. Unfortunately, years of bad science told us that fat is something you have to avoid – but it's actually a very helpful thing for weight loss! Even before we move forward with this book, we'll have to discuss exactly what "healthy fats" are, and why they're actually the good guys. To do this, we need to make a distinction between the different kinds of fat. You've probably heard of them before and it is a little bit confusing at first. We'll try to go through them as simply as possible:

Saturated fat. This is the kind you want to avoid. They're also called "solid fat" because each molecule is packed with hydrogen atoms. Simply put, it's the kind of fat that can easily cause a blockage in your body. It can raise cholesterol levels and lead to heart problems or a stroke. Saturated fat is something you can find in meat, dairy products, and other processed food items. Now, you're probably wondering: isn't the Ketogenic Diet packed with saturated fat? The answer is: not necessarily. You'll find later in the recipes given that the Ketogenic Diet promotes primarily unsaturated fat or healthy fat. While there are definitely many meat recipes in the list, most of these recipes contain healthy fat sources.

Unsaturated Fat. These are the ones dubbed as healthy fat. They're the kind of fat you find in avocado, nuts, and other ingredients you usually find in Keto-friendly recipes. They're known to lower blood cholesterol and actually come in two types: polyunsaturated and monounsaturated. Both are good for your body but the benefits slightly vary, depending on what you're consuming.

Lemon Mushrooms

Preparation Time: 10 minutes
Cooking Time: 4 minutes
Servings: 2 servings
Ingredients:

- 1 cup cremini mushrooms, sliced
- 1 teaspoon lemon zest, grated
- 1 tablespoon lemon juice
- ½ teaspoon salt
- ½ teaspoon dried thyme
- ½ cup of water
- 1 teaspoon almond butter

Directions:

1. Put all **Ingredients:** in the instant pot and stir them with the help of the spatula.
2. Then close and seal the instant pot lid.
3. Cook the mushrooms on manual mode (high pressure) for 4 minutes.
4. When the time of cooking is finished, allow the natural pressure release for 5 minutes.

Nutrition: Calories 62, Fat 4.6 Fiber 1.2 Carbs 3.5 Protein 2.7

Feta Psiti

Preparation Time: 10 minutes
Cooking Time: 6 minutes
Servings: 6 servings
Ingredients:

- 12 oz. Feta cheese
- ½ tomato, sliced
- 1 oz. bell pepper, sliced
- 1 teaspoon ground paprika
- 1 tablespoon olive oil
- 1 cup water, for cooking

Directions:

1. Sprinkle the cheese with olive oil and ground paprika and place it on the foil.
2. Then top Feta cheese with sliced tomato and bell pepper. Wrap it in the foil well.
3. After this, pour water and insert the steamer rack in the instant pot.
4. Put the wrapped cheese on the rack. Close and seal the lid.

5. Cook the cheese on manual mode (high pressure) for 6 minutes. Then make a quick pressure release.
6. Discard the foil and transfer the cheese on the serving plates.

Nutrition: calories 178, fat 14.5, fiber 0.5, carbs 4.2, protein 8.4

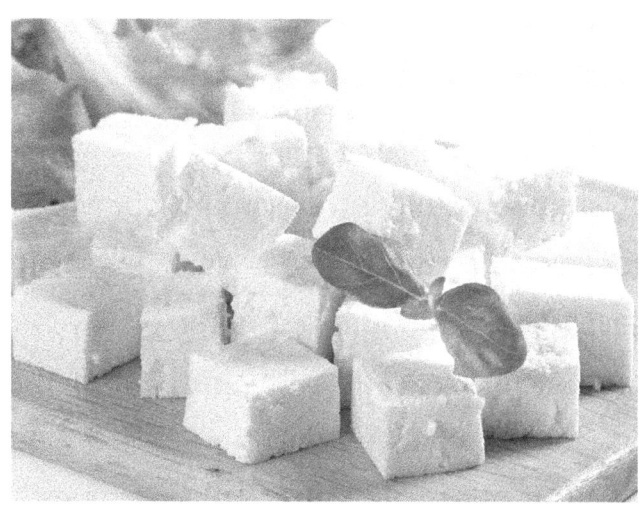

Cauliflower Queso

Preparation Time: 10 minutes
Cooking Time: 30 minutes
Servings: 5
Ingredients:
- 2 cups cauliflower, chopped
- 1/3 cup cream cheese
- ½ cup Cheddar cheese
- 1 jalapeno, chopped
- 2 oz. scallions, diced
- 1 tablespoon nutritional yeast
- 1 tablespoon olive oil
- 2 garlic cloves, diced

Directions:
1. Put chopped cauliflower, cream cheese, Cheddar cheese, jalapeno, diced scallions, nutritional yeast, olive oil, and diced garlic clove.
2. Stir the mixture well with the help of the spoon and close the lid.
3. Cook the queso for 30 minutes on saute mode. Stir meal every 5 minutes to avoid burning.

Nutrition: Calories 146 Fat 12.1 Fiber 1.9 Carbs 5 Protein 6

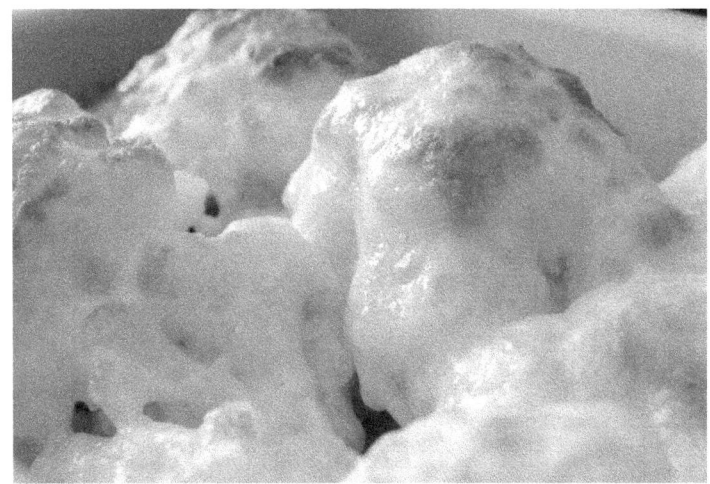

Sweet Smokies

Preparation Time: 5 minutes

Cooking Time: 15 minutes

Servings: 3 servings

Ingredients:
- 1 teaspoon Erythritol
- ½ teaspoon sesame seeds
- 2 tablespoons keto BBQ sauce
- 8 oz. cocktail sausages
- 1/3 cup chicken broth

Directions:
1. Put Erythritol, sesame seeds, BBQ sauce, and chicken broth in the instant pot.
2. Preheat the mixture on saute mode for 2 minutes.
3. Then add cocktail sausages and stir the mixture well.
4. Cook the meal for 10 minutes on saute mode. Stir the sausages every 2 minutes.

Nutrition: Calories 49 Fat 2.5 Fiber 5.7 Carbs 0.1 Protein 2.3

Rosemary Chicken Wings

Preparation Time: 10 minutes
Cooking Time: 16 minutes
Servings: 4 servings
Ingredients:
- 4 chicken wings, boneless
- 1 tablespoon olive oil
- 1 teaspoon dried rosemary
- ½ teaspoon garlic powder
- ¼ teaspoon salt

Directions:
- In the mixing bowl, mix up olive oil, dried rosemary, garlic powder, and salt.
- Then rub the chicken wings with the rosemary mixture and leave for 10 minutes to marinate.
- After this, put the chicken wings in the instant pot, add the remaining rosemary marinade and cook them on saute mode for 8 minutes from each side.

Nutrition: Calories 222 Fat 11.1 Fiber 0.2 Carbs 1.8 Protein 27.5

Classic Meatballs

Preparation Time: 20 minutes
Cooking Time: 15 minutes
Servings: 6
Ingredients:
- 7 oz. ground beef
- 7 oz. ground pork
- 1 teaspoon minced garlic
- 3 tablespoons water
- 1 teaspoon chili flakes
- 1 teaspoon dried parsley
- 1 tablespoon coconut oil
- ¼ cup beef broth

Directions:
1. In the mixing bowl, mix up ground beef, ground pork, minced garlic, water, and chili flakes, and dried parsley.
2. Make the medium size meatballs from the mixture.
3. After this, heat up coconut oil in the instant pot on saute mode.

4. Put the meatballs in the hot coconut oil in one layer and cook them for 2 minutes from each side.
5. Then add beef broth and close the lid.
6. Cook the meatballs for 10 minutes on manual mode (high pressure).
7. Then make a quick pressure release and transfer the meatballs on the plate.

Nutrition: Calories 131 Fat 5.6 Fiber 0 Carbs 0.2 Protein 18.9

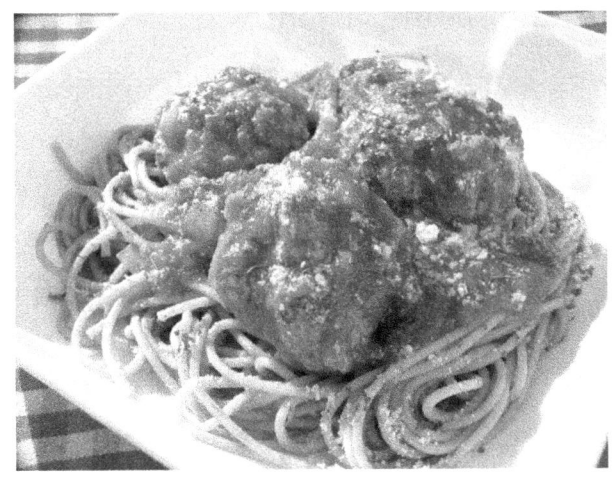

Bacon Deviled Eggs

Preparation Time: 10 minutes
Cooking Time: 15 minutes
Servings: 4
Ingredients:
- 2 eggs
- 1 teaspoon cream cheese
- 1 oz. Parmesan, grated
- ¼ teaspoon red pepper
- 1 oz. bacon, chopped
- 1 cup of water

Directions:
1. Pour water in the instant pot.
2. Add eggs and cook them for 5 minutes on manual mode (high pressure).
3. Then make a quick pressure release. Cool and peel the eggs.
4. After this, clean the instant pot bowl and put the bacon inside.
5. Cook it on saute mode for 10 minutes. Stir it from time to time to avoid burning.
6. Cut the eggs into halves.

7. Put the egg yolks in the bowl and smash them with the help of the fork.
8. Add red pepper, cooked bacon, and cream cheese. Mix up the mixture.
9. Then fill the egg whites with the bacon mixture.

Nutrition: Calories 98 Fat 7 Fiber 0.1 Carbs 1.1 Protein 7.8

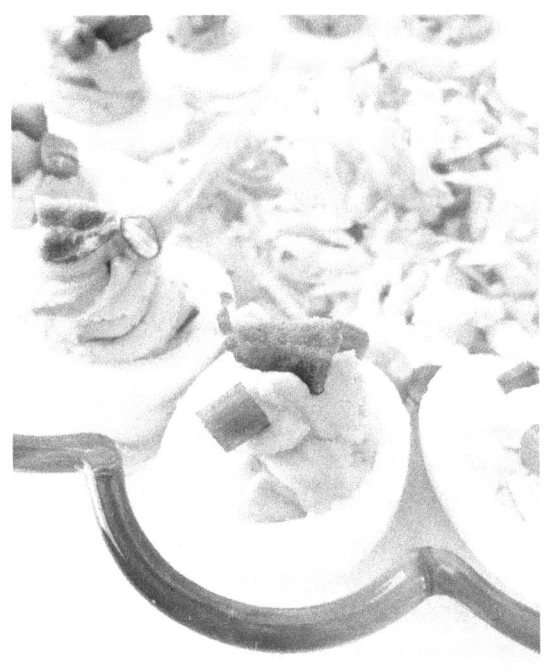

Spinach Dip

Preparation Time: 10 minutes

Cooking Time: 6 hours

Servings: 4

Ingredients:

- 2 cups spinach, chopped
- 1 cup Mozzarella, shredded
- 2 artichoke hearts, chopped
- 1 teaspoon ground ginger
- 1 teaspoon butter
- ½ teaspoon white pepper
- ½ cup heavy cream

Directions:

1. Put the spinach, artichoke hearts, and butter in the instant pot bowl.
2. Add Mozzarella, ground ginger, white pepper, and heavy cream. Stir the mixture gently.
3. Cook it in manual mode (Low pressure) for 6 hours. Then stir well and transfer in the serving bowl.

Nutrition: Calories 124 Fat 8 Fiber 4.8 Carbs 10.2 Protein 5.5

Sausage Balls

Preparation Time: 10 minutes
Cooking Time: 16 minutes
Servings: 10
Ingredients:

- 15 oz. ground pork sausage
- 1 teaspoon dried oregano
- 4 oz. Mozzarella, shredded
- 1 cup coconut flour
- 1 garlic clove, grated
- 1 teaspoon coconut oil, melted

Directions:

1. In the bowl mix up ground pork sausages, dried oregano, shredded Mozzarella, coconut flour, and garlic clove.
2. When the mixture is homogenous, make the balls.
3. After this, pour coconut oil in the instant pot.
4. Arrange the balls in the instant pot and cook them on saute mode for 8 minutes from each side.

Nutrition: Calories 310 Fat 23.2 Fiber 4.9 Carbs 10.1 Protein 16.8

BLT Dip

Preparation Time: 10 minutes
Cooking Time: 20 minutes
Servings: 3
Ingredients:
- 2 teaspoons cream cheese
- 3 oz. bacon, chopped
- 2 tablespoons sour cream
- 2 oz. Cheddar cheese, shredded
- ¼ teaspoon minced garlic
- 1 teaspoon smoked paprika
- 1 tomato, chopped
- ¼ cup lettuce, chopped

Directions:
1. Preheat the instant pot on saute mode.
2. Put the chopped bacon in the instant pot and cook it for 5 minutes. Stir it from time to time.
3. Then add cream cheese, sour cream, Cheddar cheese, garlic, smoked paprika, and tomato.
4. Close the lid and cook the dip on saute mode for 15 minutes.
5. Then stir it well and mix up with lettuce.

Nutrition: Calories 261 Fat 20.7 Fiber 0.5 Carbs 2.5 Protein 15.9

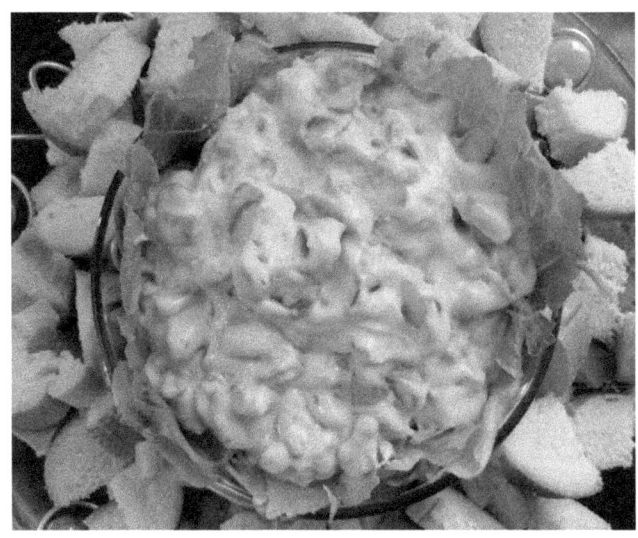

DESSERTS

Southern Apple Pie

Preparation Time: 15 minutes
Cooking Time: 40 minutes
Servings: 8 persons
Ingredients
- Crust:
- 2 cups blanched almond flour
- ½ cup butter
- ½ cup powdered Erythritol
- 1 teaspoon allspice
- Filling:
- 3 cups sliced apples
- ¼ cup melted butter
- ½ lemon, juiced
- ¼ cup powdered Erythritol
- ½ teaspoon allspice
- Topping:
- Cinnamon, as desired
- Granulated Erythritol, as desired

Directions
1. Prepare the crust; preheat oven to 375F.
2. Melt the butter in a microwave safe bowl.
3. Combine almond flour, melted butter, and remaining crust ingredients until the dough comes together.
4. Press the crust into 9-inch springform.
5. Cover the crust with parchment paper and baking balls (or rice) and bake 10 minutes.
6. In the meantime, make the filling; toss the sliced apples with juice.
7. Remove the crust from the oven. Fill with the apples in a circular pattern.
8. Combine butter, Erythritol, and allspice in a bowl.
9. Pour over the apples.
10. Bake the pie for 30 minutes.
11. Remove the pie from the oven and allow to cool.
12. Combine desired amounts of cinnamon and Erythritol.
13. Sprinkle the apples with the cinnamon mixture.
14. Slice and serve.

Nutrition Calories 123, Fat 9.2g, Carbs 4.8g, Protein 8.3g

Lemon Cheesecake

Preparation Time: 15 minutes
Cooking Time: 25 minutes
Servings: 12 persons

Ingredients

- Crust:
- 2 teaspoons granulated Erythritol
- 2 cups almond flour
- ½ cup unsalted melted butter
- ¼ cup desiccated coconut
- Filling:
- 1 tablespoon powdered gelatin
- 2 tablespoons granulated Erythritol
- ¾ cup boiling water
- ½ cup cold water
- 1lb. cream cheese
- 2 lemons, zested and juice

Directions

1. Prepare the crust; combine the crust ingredients in a large mixing bowl.
2. Stir until the dough comes together.
3. Transfer the dough into 9-inch springform.
4. Place in a fridge while you make the filling.

5. Prepare the filling; pour the water in a bowl. Sprinkle over the gelatin powder. Pour in cold water and place aside for 5 minutes.
6. Beat cream cheese, gelatin mixture, Erythritol, lemon juice and zest in a mixing bowl.
7. Pour the filling over the crust.
8. Refrigerate for 2 hours.
9. Slice and serve.

Nutrition Calories 143, Fat 9.2g, Carbs 4.8g, Protein 8.3g

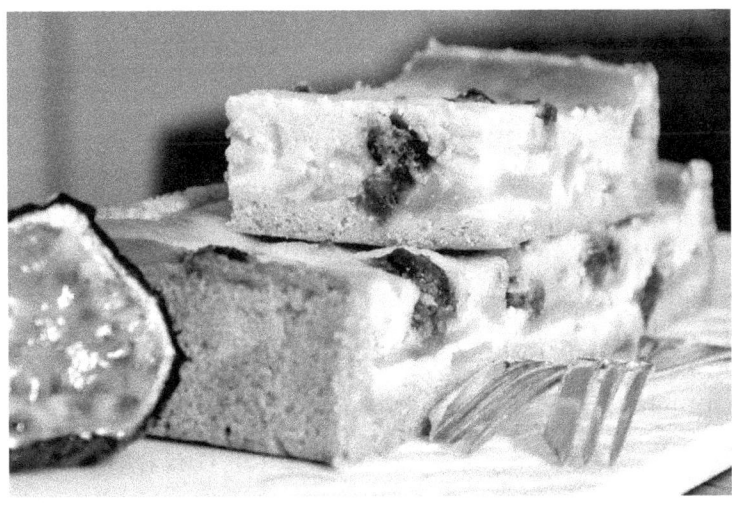

No-Guilt Chocolate Cake

Preparation Time: 15 minutes + inactive time
Cooking Time: 25 minutes
Servings: 8 persons

Ingredients

- ¾ cup butter
- 12oz. sugar-free quality dark chocolate, chopped or chocolate chips
- 1 teaspoon sugar-free vanilla extract
- 3 large eggs, room temperature
- 1 pinch salt
- ¼ cup granulated Erythritol
- 10 drops liquid Stevia

Directions

1. Preheat oven to 350F.
2. Line 8-inch springform pan with baking paper. Additionally, grease with some coconut oil for easy removal.
3. Melt butter and chopped chocolate over a double boiler.
4. Remove from the heat and pour the mixture into a large bowl.
5. Beat in vanilla and salt.

6. Beat in the eggs, one at the time, and beating well after each addition.
7. Fold in the sweetener.
8. Strain the mixture through a fine sieve into the prepared springform.
9. Gently tap the springform onto the kitchen counter.
10. Bake the cake for 25 minutes.
11. Cool the cake to room temperature and refrigerate for at least 8 hours.
12. Slice and serve, with a dollop of whipped coconut cream.

Nutrition Calories 103, Fat 9.2g, Carbs 4.8g, Protein 8.3g

Cheese Berry Pie

Preparation Time: 15 minutes
Cooking Time: 25 minutes
Servings: 8 persons
Ingredients
- Crust:
- 1 cup coconut oil, solid
- 4 large eggs
- 1 pinch salt
- 1 ½ cups softened coconut flour
- 1 tablespoon cold water
- ½ teaspoon baking powder
- Filling:
- 1 ½ cups fresh blueberries
- 2 tablespoons granulated Erythritol
- 1 cup cream cheese

Directions
1. Preheat oven to 350F.
2. Make the crust; combine coconut flour, salt, and baking powder in a bowl.
3. Work in coconut oil.
4. Add eggs, one at the time until incorporated.
5. Add water and stir until you have a smooth dough. Divide the dough into two equal parts.

6. Transfer the one part into 9-inch pie pan. Roll out the second and place aside.
7. Prepare the filling; spread cream cheese over the crust.
8. Toss the blueberries with the Erythritol and spread over the cheese.
9. Top the pie with the remaining dough.
10. Bake the pie for 25 minutes.
11. Cool the pie on a rack for 10 minutes.
12. Slice and serve.

Nutrition Calories 143, Fat 9.2g, Carbs 4.8g, Protein 8.3g

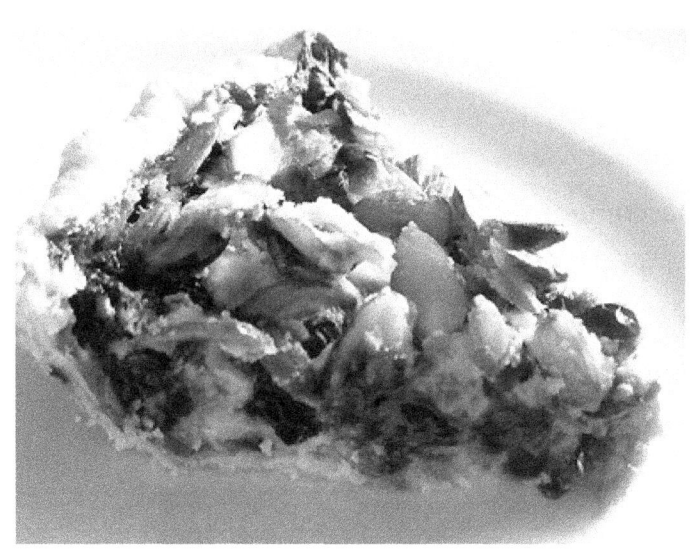

The Best Cookies

Preparation Time: 15 minutes
Cooking Time: 10 minutes
Servings: 16 persons

Ingredients

- 1/3 cup coconut oil
- 1 ½ teaspoon sugar-free vanilla extract
- 1 medium egg
- 1 pinch salt
- 3 tablespoons granulated Erythritol
- 1 cup almond flour
- 2 tablespoons coconut flour
- ½ teaspoon cinnamon
- 1/3 cup sugar-free quality dark chocolate chips

Directions

1. Preheat oven to 350F. Line baking sheet with a parchment paper.
2. In a mixing bowl, beat egg with vanilla and Erythritol.
3. Melt the coconut oil and fold into the egg mixture.
4. Fold in the remaining ingredients and stir until the dough comes together.
5. Let the dough stand for 5 minutes.
6. Scoop the dough with a cookie scoop, onto the baking sheet.

7. Press gently with the back of your spoon to flatten.
8. Bake the cookies for 10 minutes.
9. Cool briefly on a wire rack before serving.
10. Serve with a cup of almond milk and enjoy.

Nutrition Calories 143, Fat 9.2g, Carbs 4.8g, Protein 8.3

Salty Caramel Cake

Preparation Time: 15 minutes
Cooking Time: 25 minutes
Servings: 10 persons

Ingredients
- 2 cups blanched almond flour
- 3 tablespoons coconut flour
- 2 tablespoons vanilla whey protein powder
- ¾ tablespoon baking powder
- 1/3 cup unsalted butter
- 1 pinch salt
- ½ cup granulated Erythritol
- 3 large eggs, room temperature
- 1 teaspoon sugar-free vanilla extract
- ½ cup unsweetened almond milk
- 2 cups sugar-free caramel sauce
- Sea salt flakes, for sprinkle

Directions
1. Preheat oven to 325F.
2. Line 2 8-inch spring form pans with baking paper.
3. In a mixing bowl, combine all the dry ingredients, except the sweetener.
4. In a separate bowl, cream butter, and Erythritol.

5. Beat in eggs, one at the time, followed by vanilla and almond milk
6. Fold the liquid ingredients into the dry ones.
7. Divide the batter between two spring form pans.
8. Bake the sponges for 25 minutes or until the inserted toothpick comes out clean.
9. Place the sponges aside to cool.
10. Spread 1 ½ cups of the caramel sauce over one sponge. Top with the second sponge.
11. Pour the remaining caramel over the top.
12. Sprinkle the caramel with salt flakes. Refrigerate the cake for 1 hour. Slice and serve.

Nutrition Calories 143, Fat 9.2g, Carbs 4.8g, Protein 8.3g

Luscious Red Velvet Cake

Preparation Time: 15 minutes + inactive time

Cooking Time: 25 minutes

Servings: 10 persons

Ingredients

- Cake:
- 1 cup granulated Erythritol
- ½ cup coconut flour
- ½ cup Swerve
- 2 tablespoons raw cocoa powder
- 6 large eggs, separated
- ½ cup melted and cooled butter
- 2 tablespoons crème Fraiche
- 1 tablespoon powdered red food coloring
- 1 teaspoon white vinegar
- 1 teaspoon sugar-free vanilla
- Frosting:
- 4oz. cream cheese
- 4 tablespoons softened unsalted butter
- 2 cups Swerve
- 1 tablespoon heavy cream
- ½ teaspoon sugar-free vanilla extract

Directions

1. Preheat oven to 350F.

2. Line 9-inch springform with a baking paper and grease with some coconut oil.
3. Combine all the dry ingredients in a large mixing bowl.
4. In a separate bowl, beat eggs, butter, crème Fraiche, vinegar, and vanilla.
5. Fold the liquid ingredients into the dry ones and stir until smooth.
6. Pour the batter into the springform.
7. Bake the cake for 25-30 minutes or until the inserted toothpick comes out clean.
8. Make the frosting; beat cream cheese and butter in a bowl until fluffy.
9. Add sugar and heavy cream.
10. Beat until smooth.
11. Remove the cake from the springform once completely cold.
12. Top with the frosting.
13. Refrigerate the cake for 30 minutes.
14. Slice and serve.

Nutrition Calories 143, Fat 9.2g, Carbs 4.8g, Protein 8.3g

Southern Pecan Pie

Preparation Time: 15 minutes

Cooking Time: 50 minutes

Servings: 10 persons

Ingredients

- Crust:
- 3 cups blanched almond flour
- 4 large eggs, room temperature
- ½ cup unsalted melted butter
- ½ cup Swerve
- 1 good pinch salt
- Filling:
- 1 cup coconut oil or butter
- ¾ cup golden Swerve
- ½ cup granulated Erythritol
- 1 ½ tablespoon sugar-free maple syrup
- 4 large eggs, room temperature
- 1 ½ cup pecans, chopped
- ¾ cup pecan halves
- 2 teaspoon vanilla-bourbon extract

Directions

1. Preheat oven to 325F.
2. Grease 10-inch cast iron skillet with butter.

3. In a large mixing bowl, combine the crust ingredients until the smooth dough is formed.
4. Transfer the dough into the skillet and press so you cover the bottom and sides.
5. Prepare the filling; melt butter in a saucepot and fold in sweeteners and sugar-free maple syrup. Stir until the sweeteners are dissolved. Place aside to cool.
6. Beat the eggs with cold syrup until fluffy. Fold in pecan pieces.
7. Pour the sauce into the crust.
8. Top with pecan halves.
9. Cover the pie with an aluminum foil. Bake the pie for 40 minutes.
10. Cool before slicing and serving.

Nutrition Calories 143, Fat 9.2g, Carbs 4.8g, Protein 8.3g

Pepperoni Pizza Cups

Preparation Time: 10 minutes
Cooking Time: 8 minutes
Servings: 24
Ingredients:
- 24 mini mozzarella balls
- 24 small basil leaves
- 24 pepperoni slices in sandwich style
- sliced black olives, optional
- 1 small jar pizza sauce

Directions:
1. Preheat oven to 400°F, in the meantime take each pepperonis slice and make half inch cuts at the edges, giving it a shape of circular cross. Make sure that the center remains uncut.
2. Take the muffin pan, grease it with oil and adjust all the prepared pepperonis into it.
3. Place in the preheated oven and bake for 5 minutes or until the edges get crispy and the color is still red.
4. Remove from the oven and set aside to cool for 5 minutes, then transfer to the paper towel, so that the excess oil gets absorbed.
5. Clean the pan with a paper towel and place the cups again into the pan.

6. Put basil leaf in the center of each pepperoni, then add ½ tsp pizza sauce, mozzarella ball and olive slice in the end.
7. Bake in the oven for another 3 minutes or until the time when cheese starts melting.
8. Remove from the oven and set aside to cool for 5 minutes before transferring to the serving plate.

Nutrition: Calories: 70 Fat: 6 Carbohydrates: 1 Protein: 32

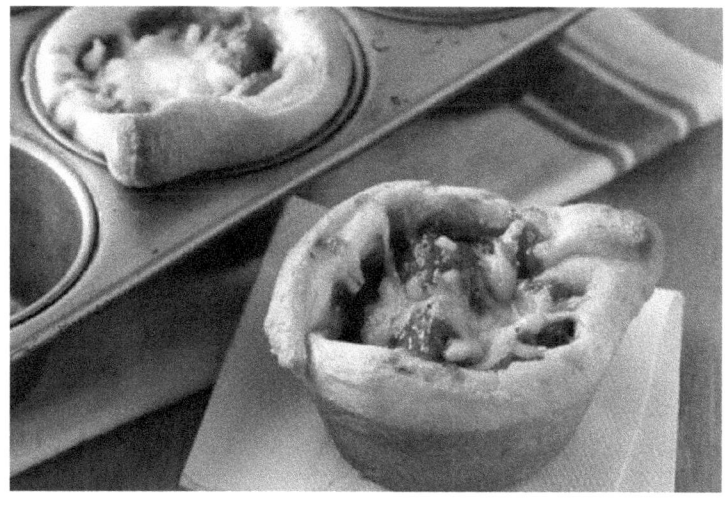

White Pizza Frittata

Preparation Time: 10 minutes
Cooking Time: 30 minutes
Servings: 8
Ingredients:

- 5 ounces mozzarella cheese
- 9 ounces bag frozen spinach
- 12 large eggs
- 4 tablespoons olive oil
- 1 ounce pepperoni
- ¼ teaspoon nutmeg
- 1 teaspoon minced garlic
- ½ cup grated parmesan cheese
- ½ cup fresh ricotta cheese
- Salt and pepper

Directions:

1. Preheat oven to 375°F in the meantime you are getting things ready.
2. Take the frozen spinach and microwave it for 3 minutes or until defrosted.
3. Squeeze the spinach using your hands to drain the excess water.

4. Take a large bowl, crack all the eggs into it, and add the spices and olive oil. Whisk them together until well blended.
5. Add the spinach, parmesan cheese and ricotta cheese and make sure that the spinach is added in small pieces. Mix together all the ingredients to prepare a good mixture.
6. Transfer the mixture to the skillet, sprinkle cheese at the top, and then add the pepperoni.
7. Place in the preheated oven and bake for 30 minutes or until the time you are satisfied.
8. Remove from the oven once baked properly and serve with a keto sauce you love.

Nutrition: Calories: 301 Fat: 25 Carbohydrates: 3 Protein: 18

Walnut Cookies

Preparation Time: 10 minutes
Cooking Time: 15 minutes
Servings: 16
Ingredients:
- 1/4 cup coconut flour
- 8 tablespoon butter
- 1/2 cup erythritol
- 1 cup walnuts
- 1 teaspoon ground nutmeg
- 1 teaspoon vanilla extract

Directions:
1. Preheat oven to 325°F, and in the meantime take the baking sheet and line it with parchment paper.
2. Grind the walnuts in a food processor and keep pulsing until they are well ground.
3. Add the vanilla extract, erythritol, nutmeg and coconut floor to the ground walnuts in the food processer. Pulse again until all the ingredients are blended.
4. Put butter in the food processer in the form of small pieces and pulse until you get a soft and smooth mixture.

5. Make 16 balls on the baking sheet with the help of a cookie scooper and use your hands to press them to give them a cookie shape.
6. Place in the preheated oven and bake for 15 minutes or until you find the cookies well baked.
7. Remove from the oven once baked, set them aside for 15-20 minutes to cool.
8. Sprinkle some additional nutmeg over the delicious walnut cookies if you like before you serve them.

Nutrition: Calories: 340 Fat: 26 Carbohydrates: 3 Protein: 19

Fathead Sausage Rolls

Preparation Time: 15 minutes
Cooking Time: 30 minutes
Servings: 6
Ingredients:

- 1 egg
- Pre-shredded grated mozzarella cheese (170g)
- 6 sausages (500g)
- Almond flour (85g)
- 2 tablespoon cream cheese full fat
- 1 teaspoon onion flakes
- Pinch salt to taste
- Onion flakes to garnish

Directions:

1. Preheat oven to 350°F and in the meantime remove the casing of all sausages and discard them.
2. Transfer the sausages to the lined baking pan.
3. Place in the preheated oven and bake for around 10 minutes.
4. Take a medium size bowl, add almond flour and cheese to it. Mix them together completely.
5. Add the cream cheese to the mixture, whisk until fully blended.

6. Microwave the mixture for 60 seconds and remove, then stir a bit and microwave again for 30 seconds, remove and stir.
7. Crack the egg into the mixture, add the onion flakes and salt. Keep mixing and pressing with a spoon to prepare a soft dough.
8. Spread the dough over a parchment paper, place another parchment paper at the top, press with your hands and give it a shape of rectangle using a roller. Make sure that you roll evenly on all sides to prepare a good fat head pastry.
9. Cut a piece of the prepared fat head pastry and wrap it around a sausage. Repeat it with all the remaining sausages.
10. Cut the wrapped sausage rolls in your desired sizes, transfer them to the baking sheet and sprinkle the sesame seeds over the top if you prefer.
11. Heat the oven to 425°F, and bake for 15 minutes or until you get a golden brown look.
12. Remove from the oven once baked, and serve with your favorite keto sauce.

Nutrition: Calories: 470 Fat: 39 Carbohydrates: 5 Protein: 26

Chia Seed Crackers

Preparation Time: 5 minutes
Cooking Time: 35 minutes
Servings: 8
Ingredients:
- 1/2 cup ground chia seeds
- 1 1/2 cups water
- 1/4 teaspoon paprika
- 1/4 teaspoon black pepper
- 1/4 teaspoon dried oregano
- 3 oz. shredded cheddar cheese
- 2 tablespoon almond meal
- 1/4 teaspoon garlic powder
- 4 tablespoon olive oil
- 1/4 teaspoon salt

Directions:
1. Preheat oven to 375°F and in the meantime take a large bowl and mix oregano, garlic powder, almond meal, paprika, chia seeds, salt and pepper. Mix together until all the ingredients are well combined.
2. Take the olive oil and pour into the mixture. Whisk until fully blended.
3. Pour water into the mixture and keep mixing until you see the smoothness.

4. Add the shredded cheddar cheese, mix it well with the mixture using a spatula and then prepare the dough kneading with your hands.
5. Spread the dough on a parchment paper in the baking sheet, cover with another parchment paper from the top and make it 0.125 inch thin with the help of a roller.
6. Place in the preheated oven and bake for 30 minutes.
7. Cut into the shapes you like after removing from the oven and place in the oven again to bake for 5 minutes more or until the time you are satisfied.
8. Remove from the oven once properly baked and transfer to the wire rack to cool before you serve the delicious chia seed crackers.

Nutrition: Calories: 120 Fat: 13 Carbohydrates: 2 Protein: 4

Cheesy Biscuits

Preparation Time: 20 minutes
Cooking Time: 20 minutes
Servings: 9
Ingredients:
- 4 eggs
- 2 cups almond flour
- 2 ½ cups shredded cheddar cheese
- 1/4 cup half-and-half
- 1 tablespoon baking powder

Directions:
1. Preheat oven to 350°F and get the baking sheet ready by lining it with parchment paper.
2. Take a large bowl and mix the baking powder and almond flour in that.
3. Add cheddar cheese to the mixture and mix until well combined.
4. Take a small bowl, add half and half and also crack the eggs into it. Mix well until fully blended.
5. Add the eggs mixture to the flour mixture and keep whisking with the help of a spatula to prepare a smooth batter.
6. Take portions of the batter using a scoop and put them on the baking sheet. Make sure that you take

the portions in even sizes and flatten them a bit from the top.
7. Place in the preheated oven and bake for 20 minutes or until the time you get a golden-brown look.
8. Remove from the oven once baked and transfer to the wire rack to cool before serving.

Nutrition: Calories: 320 Fat: 27 Carbohydrates: 8 Protein: 15

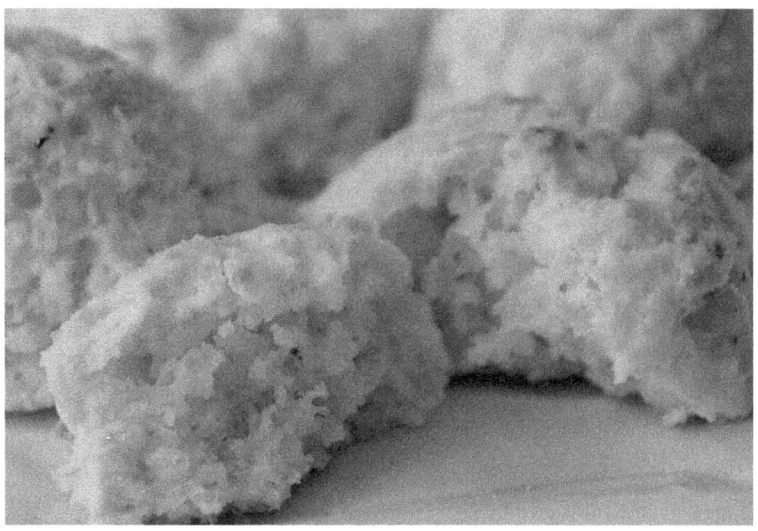

Chicken rolls with pesto

Preparation Time: 20 minutes
Cooking Time: 30 minutes
Servings: 1
Ingredients:
- Tablespoon pine nuts
- Yeast tablets
- Garlic cloves (chopped)
- Fresh basil
- Olive oil
- Chicken breast ready to slice:

Directions
1. Season with salt and pepper.
2. Place each piece of the chicken breast between 2 pieces of plastic wrap. 7 Roll in a frying pan or pasta until the chicken breasts grow out.
3. 0.6 cm thick.
4. Remove the plastic wrap, then apply pesto to the chicken.
5. Roll up the chicken breast and tie it with the cocktail skewers.
6. Season with salt and pepper.
7. Dissolve the coconut oil in the pan and use a high temperature to brown all sides of the chicken skin.

8. Place the chicken rolls on a baking sheet, place in the oven, and bake for 15 to 20 minutes, until cooked.
9. Slice it diagonally and serve it with other pesto sauce.
10. It was served with tomato salad.

Nutrition: Calories: 150, Sodium: 33 mg, Dietary Fibre: 1.6 g, Total Fat: 4.3 g, Total Carbs: 15.4 g, Protein: 1.6 g.

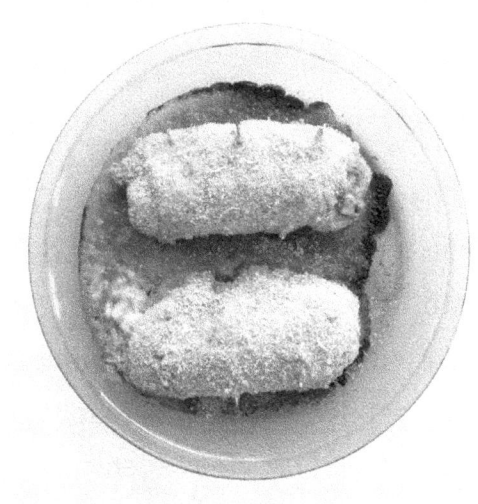

Sweet and sour sauce:

Preparation Time: 10 minutes
Cooking Time: 10 minutes
Servings: 1
Ingredients
- Apple cider vinegar
- 1/2 tablespoon tomato paste
- A teaspoon of coconut amino acid
- Bamboo spoon
- Water treatment
- Chopped vegetables.

Directions
1. Mix kudzu powder with five tablespoons of cold water to make a paste.
2. Then put all the other spices in the pot, then add the kudzu paste.
3. Melt coconut oil in a pan and fry onions.
4. Add green pepper, cabbage, cabbage and bean sprouts, then cook until the vegetables are tender.
5. Add pineapple and cashew nuts and mix a few times.
6. Just pour a little spice into the pot.

Nutrition: Calories: 3495, Sodium: 33 mg, Dietary Fibre: 1.4 g, Total Fat: 4.5 g, Total Carbs: 16.5 g, Protein: 1.7 g.

Coconut Curry Cauliflower Soup

Preparation Time: 10 minutes

Cooking Time: 25 minutes

Servings: 10

Ingredients:

- 2 tablespoons olive oil
- 1 onion, chopped
- 3 tablespoons yellow curry paste
- 2 heads cauliflower, sliced into florets
- 32 oz. vegetable broth
- 1 cup coconut milk
- Minced fresh cilantro

Directions:

1. In a pan over medium heat, add the oil.
2. Cook onion for 3 minutes.
3. Stir in the curry paste and cook for 2 minutes.
4. Add the cauliflower florets.
5. Pour in the broth.
6. Increase the heat to high and bring to a boil.
7. Lower the heat to medium.
8. Cook while covered for 20 minutes.
9. Add the coconut milk and cook for an additional minute.
10. Puree in a blender.

11. Garnish with fresh cilantro.

Nutrition: Calories 138 Total Fat 11.8g Saturated Fat 5.6g Cholesterol 0mg Sodium 430mg Total Carbohydrate 6.4g Dietary Fiber 3g Total Sugars 2.8g Protein 3.6g Potassium 318mg

Chocolate Cake with Vanilla Glaze

Preparation Time: 20 minutes
Cooking Time: 40 minutes
Servings: 6
Ingredients:

- ½ cup almond flour
- 4 tbsp butter
- 3 tbsp stevia powder
- 5 large egg yolks
- 1 tsp agar powder
- ½ tsp salt
- 2 tbsp cocoa powder
- 1 tsp chocolate extract, unsweetened
- For the glaze:
- 1 cup Mascarpone cheese
- 5 large egg whites
- 2 tbsp swerve
- 2 tsp vanilla extract
- Dark chocolate chips, optional

Directions:

1. Plug in the instant pot and pour 1 cup of water in the stainless-steel insert. Line a fitting springform pan with some parchment paper and set aside.

2. In a large mixing bowl, combine egg yolks and butter. Beat with a hand mixer for 2-3 minutes, or until well combined. Add stevia, agar powder, salt, and cocoa, Beat again for 2 minutes. Finally, add almond flour and beat again until fully combined.
3. Pour the mixture in the springform pan and gently flatten the surface with a spatula.
4. Set the trivet on the bottom of your pot and place the pan on the top. Close the lid and adjust the steam release handle. Press the "Manual" button and set the timer for 40 minutes. Cook on "High" pressure.
5. Meanwhile, combine all glaze ingredients and remaining egg whites in a large mixing bowl. Beat until well combined and set aside.
6. When you hear the cooker's end signal, perform a quick pressure release and open the pot. Transfer the pan to a wire rack and let it cool for 10 minutes.
7. Top the cake with glaze and spread evenly. Add ½ cup of water to the pot and return the pan on top of the trivet. Close the lid and adjust the steam release handle. Cook for 1 minutes on the "Manual" mode.
8. When done, perform a quick pressure release and open the pot.
9. Chill to a room temperature and refrigerate for 20 minutes before serving.

10. Optionally, top with some dark chocolate chips for some extra flavor.

Nutrition: Calories 263 Total Fats: 21.5g Net Carbs: 3.6g Protein: 12.3g Fiber: 1.6g

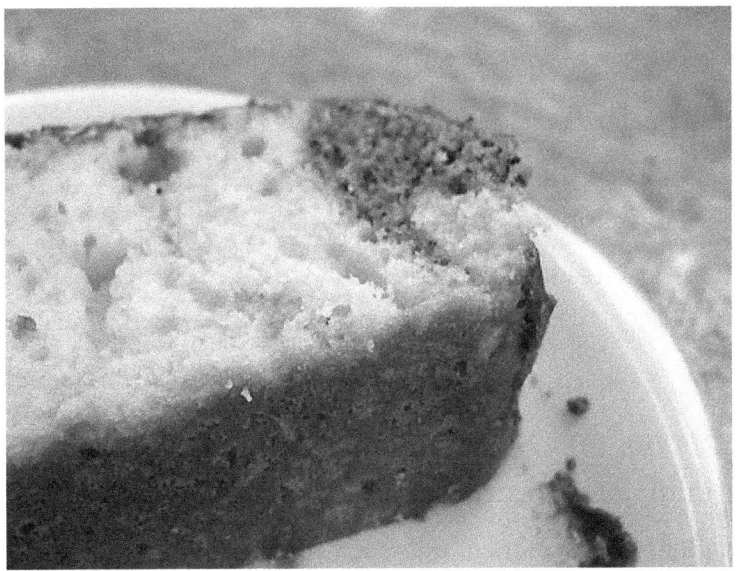

Rum Truffles

Preparation Time: 20 minutes
Cooking Time: 30 minutes
Servings: 5
Ingredients:
- ½ cup dark chocolate chips, melted
- 1 cup heavy cream
- ¼ cup granulated stevia
- ¼ tsp xanthan gum
- 3 egg yolks
- ½ cup whipped cream
- Spices:
- ½ tsp rum extract
- ¼ tsp cinnamon, ground
- ½ tsp stevia powder

Directions:
1. In a mixing bowl, combine egg yolks, granulated stevia, and xanthan gum. Using a hand mixer, beat until well incorporated. Add heavy cream, melted chocolate chips, rum extract, cinnamon, and stevia powder. Beat for 1 more minute and then pour into oven-safe ramekins. Wrap the top of each ramekin with aluminum foil and set aside.

2. Plug in your instant pot and pour 1 cup of water in the stainless-steel insert. Position a trivet on the bottom and place ramekins on top. Close the lid and adjust the steam release handle. Press the "Manual" button and set the timer for 30 minutes. Cook on "High" pressure.
3. When you hear the cooker's end signal, release the pressure naturally. Open the pot and top with whipped cream and powdered stevia before serving.

Nutrition: Calories 208 Total Fats: 18.5g Net Carbs: 9.4g Protein: 3.2g Fiber: 0.1g

Mint Cake

Preparation Time: 15 minutes
Cooking Time: 45 minutes
Servings: 8
Ingredients:
- For the layers:
- 1 cup almond flour
- 1 cup coconut flour
- 1 tbsp stevia powder
- ¼ cup whole milk
- 3 tbsp butter
- 5 large eggs
- 1 tsp vanilla extract
- ½ tsp salt
- For the filling:
- ¼ cup butter
- ½ cup cream cheese
- 2 tsp stevia powder
- 1 tsp mint extract

Directions:
1. In a large mixing bowl, combine almond flour, coconut flour, stevia powder, and salt. Mix until combined and set aside.

2. In a separate bowl, combine eggs, butter, milk, and vanilla extract. Using a hand mixer, beat until fluffy and then gradually add to dry ingredients. Mix until all well incorporated. Set aside.
3. In another bowl, combine all filling ingredients. With a paddle attachment on, beat until well combined and set aside.
4. Pour 1 cup of water in the stainless steel of your instant pot. Line a fitting springform pan with some parchment paper. Set the trivet on the bottom of the pot and place the pan on top. Pour half of the layer mixture in the pan and close the lid. Adjust the steam release handle and press the "Manual" button. Set the timer for 20 minutes and cook on "High" pressure,
5. When you hear the cooker's end signal, perform a quick pressure release and open the pot. Transfer the layer to a wire rack to cool. Repeat the process with the remaining mixture.
6. When the second layer is done, spread the filling over and top with the remaining layer. Close the lid of your pot and adjust the steam release handle. Press the "Manual" button and set the timer for 5 minutes on "High" pressure.
7. When done, perform a quick pressure release and open the pot.

8. Chill to a room temperature before serving and optionally, garnish with some fresh mint.

Nutrition: Calories 398 Total Fats: 33.8g Net Carbs: 6.6g Protein: 10.5g Fiber: 7.5g

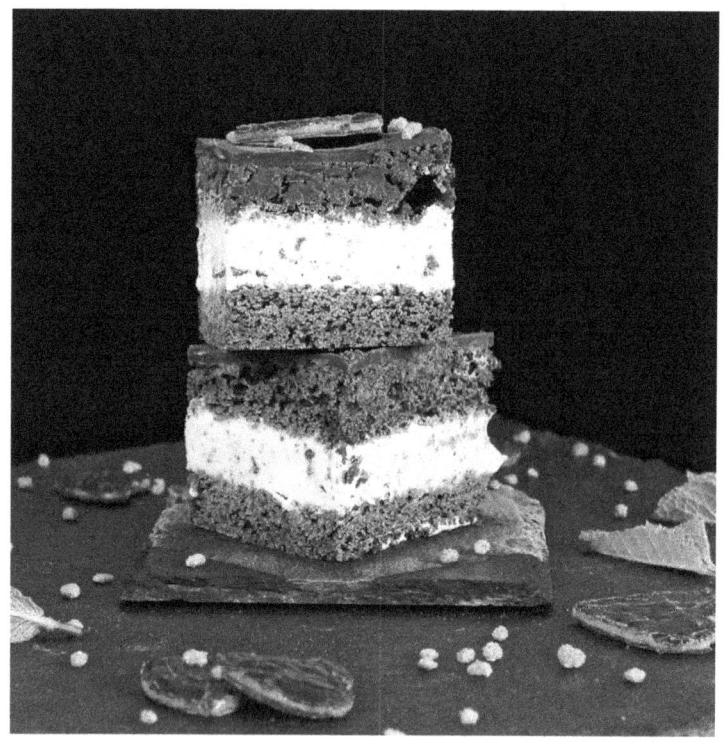

Vanilla Cherry Panna Cotta

Preparation Time: 5 minutes
Cooking Time: 10 minutes
Servings: 2
Ingredients:

- For the vanilla layer:
- 1 cup heavy whipping cream
- 2 tbsp whole milk
- 1 tsp agar powder
- ½ tsp vanilla extract
- 1 tbsp walnuts, roughly chopped
- For the cherry layer:
- 1 cup heavy whipping cream
- 1 tsp agar powder
- 1 tbsp almonds, roughly chopped
- 2 tsp cherry extract

Directions:

1. Plug in the instant pot and combine all vanilla layer ingredients in the stainless-steel insert. Press the "Saute" button and stir constantly. Bring it to a light simmer and then press "Cancel" button. Transfer to a large bowl and set aside.

2. Clean the pot and pat-dry with a kitchen paper. Now, add all cherry layer ingredients and stir well. Again, bring it to a light simmer, stirring constantly.
3. Pour about ½-inch thick vanilla layer in a medium-sized glass. Now, add the second layer of the cherry mixture. Repeat the process until you have used both mixtures.
4. Optionally, garnish with some fresh mint and refrigerate for at least 1 hour before serving.

Nutrition: Calories 467 Total Fats: 48.7g Net Carbs: 4.6g Protein: 4.5gFiber: 0.8g

Keto Berry Pancakes

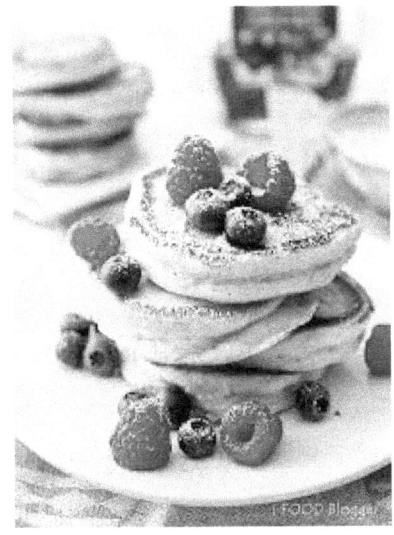

Preparation Time: 5 minutes

Cooking Time: 15 minutes

Servings: 10

Ingredients:

- 1/2 cup almond flour
- 4 pieces large eggs
- 4 ounces cream cheese (softened)
- 1 teaspoon lemon zest
- 1 tablespoon butter (for frying)
- 1 tablespoon butter (for topping)
- 1/2 cup of frozen berries

Directions:

1. In a mixing bowl, put in almond flour, eggs, cream cheese, and lemon zest. Whisk until the batter is well combined.
2. In a skillet over medium heat, melt the butter for frying.
3. Scoop about 3 tablespoons of batter and pour it on the skillet. Cook the pancake for about 2 minutes or until it turns golden.
4. Flip the pancake to its other side and cook it for another 2 minutes.
5. Transfer the cooked pancake to a plate. Continue cooking the rest of the batter.
6. Serve the pancakes topped with berries.

Nutrition: Calories: 110 Carbs: 2 g Fats: 10 g Proteins: 4 g Fiber: 1 g

Mocha Pots de Crème

Preparation Time: 10 minutes
Cooking Time: 15 minutes
Servings: 4
Ingredients:

- 2 large eggs, separated
- 1 cup coconut milk, full-fat
- ¾ cup heavy cream
- 2 tbsp cocoa powder, unsweetened
- 3 tbsp brewed espresso
- 3 tbsp stevia powder
- Spices:
- ¼ tsp salt
- 1 tsp vanilla extract

Directions:

1. In a small bowl, whisk together eggs, cocoa powder, espresso, stevia powder, vanilla, and salt. Set aside.
2. Plug in the instant pot and press the "Saute" button. Pour in the coconut milk and heavy cream. Give it a good stir and warm up.
3. Press the "Cancel" button and slowly pour the warm milk mixture over the egg mixture, whisking constantly.

4. Divide the mixture between 4 ramekins and loosely cover with aluminum foil.
5. Position a trivet at the bottom of your pot and pour in 2 cups of water. Gently place the ramekins on top and seal the lid.
6. Set the steam release handle to the "Sealing" position and press the "Manual" button.
7. Cook for 15 minutes.
8. When done, perform a quick pressure release and open the lid. Remove the ramekins and transfer to a wire rack. Cool to a room temperature and then refrigerate for about an hour.

Nutrition: Calories 257 Total Fats: 25.5g Net Carbs: 3.5g Protein: 5.5g Fiber: 2.1g

Lemon Cake with Berry Syrup

Preparation Time: 15 minutes
Cooking Time: 30 minutes
Servings: 8
Ingredients:
- For the cake:
- 3 cups almond flour
- 3 tbsp stevia powder
- ¼ cup coconut milk, full-fat
- 1 tbsp coconut cream
- ¼ cup butter, softened
- 5 large eggs
- ¼ tsp salt
- 3 tsp baking powder
- 2 tsp lemon extract
- For the syrup:
- ¼ cup raspberries
- ¼ cup blueberries
- 1 tbsp lemon juice, freshly squeeze
- ¼ cup granulated stevia

Directions:
1. In a large mixing bowl, combine together almond flour, stevia powder, baking powder, and salt.

2. Mix well and add eggs, one at the time, beating constantly.
3. Now add coconut milk, coconut cream, butter, and lemon extract. Using a paddle attachment beat for 3 minutes on medium speed.
4. Grease a small cake pan with some oil and line with parchment paper. Pour the mixture in it and tightly wrap with aluminum foil.
5. Plug in the instant pot and set the trivet at the bottom of the inner pot. Place the cake pan on top and pour in one cup of water.
6. Seal the lid and set the steam release handle to the "Sealing" position. Press the "Manual" button and cook for 25 minutes.
7. When done, perform a quick pressure release and open the lid. Carefully remove the pan and set aside.
8. Now press the "Saute" button. Add berries and pour in one cup of water and granulated stevia. Gently simmer for 5-6 minutes, stirring constantly.
9. Finally, add agar powder and give it a good stir. Cook until the mixture thickens.
10. Pour the syrup over chilled cake and refrigerate for 2 hours before serving.

Nutrition: Calories 186 Total Fats: 16g Net Carbs: 3.8g Protein: 6.4gFiber: 1.3g

Easy Rum Cheesecake

Preparation Time: 15minutes
Cooking Time: 15 minutes
Servings: 10
Ingredients:
- 2 cups almond flour
- 4 large eggs, separated
- ¼ cup coconut cream
- 2 tbsp almond butter
- ¼ cup cocoa powder, unsweetened
- ¼ cup swerve
- 3 tsp baking powder
- 3 cups Mascarpone
- 1 cup plain Greek yogurt
- 2-3 drops stevia
- Spices:
- 2 tsp rum extract
- ½ tsp cinnamon powder

Directions:
1. Plug in the instant pot and position a trivet. Pour in one cup of water in the stainless-steel insert and set aside.
2. Beat egg whites and swerve with a hand mixer until light foam appears. Add egg yolks, coconut cream,

almond butter, baking powder, and cocoa powder, beating constantly.
3. Finally, add almond flour and continue to beat until completely combined.
4. Pour the mixture into lightly greased cake pan and cook for 15 minutes on the "Manual" mode.
5. When done, perform a quick pressure release and open the lid. Remove the cake from the pan and cool for a while.
6. Now combine Mascarpone and Greek yogurt. Add rum extract, cinnamon powder, and stevia. Using a hand mixer, mix well until completely combined.
7. Pour the mixture over the crust and refrigerate for a couple of hours before slicing.

Nutrition: Calories 247 Total Fats: 18.1g Net Carbs: 5.6gProtein: 15.6g Fiber: 1.7g

Lemon Vegan Cake

Preparation Time: 10 minutes
Cooking Time: 10 minutes
Servings: 3
Ingredients:
- 1 cup of pitted dates
- 2-1/2 cups pecans
- 1-1/2 cup agave
- 3 avocados, halved & pitted
- 3 cups of cauliflower rice, prepared
- 1 lemon juice and zest
- ½ lemon extract
- 1-1/2 cups pineapple, crushed
- 1-1/2 teaspoon vanilla extract
- Pinch of cinnamon
- 1-1/2 cups of dairy-free yogurt

Directions:
1. Line your baking sheet with parchment paper.
2. Pulse the pecans in your food processor.
3. Add the agave and dates. Pulse for a minute.
4. Transfer this mix to the baking sheet. Wipe the bowl of your processor.

5. Bring together the pineapple, agave, avocados, cauliflower, lemon juice, and zest in your food processor. Get a smooth mixture.
6. Now add the lemon extract, cinnamon, and vanilla extract. Pulse.
7. Pour this mix into your pan, on the crust.
8. Refrigerate for 5 hours minimum.
9. Take out the cake and keep it at room temperature for 20 minutes.
10. Take out the cake's outer ring.
11. Whisk together the vanilla extract, agave, and yogurt in a bowl.
12. Pour on your cake.

Nutrition: Calories 688 Carbohydrates 100g Fat 28g Protein 9g Sugar 40g

Dark Chocolate Granola Bars

Preparation Time: 10 minutes

Cooking Time: 25 minutes

Servings: 12

Ingredients:

- 1 cup tart cherries, dried
- 2 cups buckwheat
- ¼ cup of flaxseed
- 1 cup of walnuts
- 2 eggs
- 1 teaspoon of salt
- ¼ cup dark cocoa powder
- 2/3 cup honey
- ½ cup dark chocolate chips
- 1 teaspoon of vanilla

Directions:

1. Preheat your oven to 350 degrees F.
2. Apply cooking spray lightly on your baking pan.
3. Pulse together the walnuts, wheat, tart cherries, salt, and flaxseed in your food processor. Everything should be chopped fine.

4. Whisk together the honey, eggs, vanilla, and cocoa powder in a bowl.
5. Add the wheat mix to your bowl. Stir to combine well.
6. Include the chocolate chips. Stir again.
7. Now pour this mixture into your baking dish.
8. Sprinkle some chocolate chips and tart cherries.
9. Bake for 25 minutes. Set aside for cooling before serving.

Nutrition: Calories 364Carbohydrates 37gCholesterol 60mgFat 20gProtein 6gSugar 22gFiber 4gSodium 214mg

Blueberry Crisp

Preparation Time: 5 minutes

Cooking Time: 30 minutes

Servings: 4

Ingredients:

- ¼ cups pecans, chopped
- 1 cup buckwheat
- ½ teaspoon ginger
- 1 teaspoon of cinnamon
- 2 tablespoons olive oil
- ¼ teaspoon nutmeg
- 1 lb. blueberries
- 1 teaspoon of honey

Directions:

1. Preheat your oven to 350 degrees F.
2. Grease your baking dish.
3. Whisk together the pecans, wheat, oil, spices, and honey in a bowl.
4. Add the berries to your pan. Layer the topping on your berries.
5. Bake for 30 minutes at 350 F.

Nutrition: Calories 327 Carbohydrates 35g Fat 19g Protein 4g Sugar 14g Fiber 5g Sodium 2mg Potassium 197mg

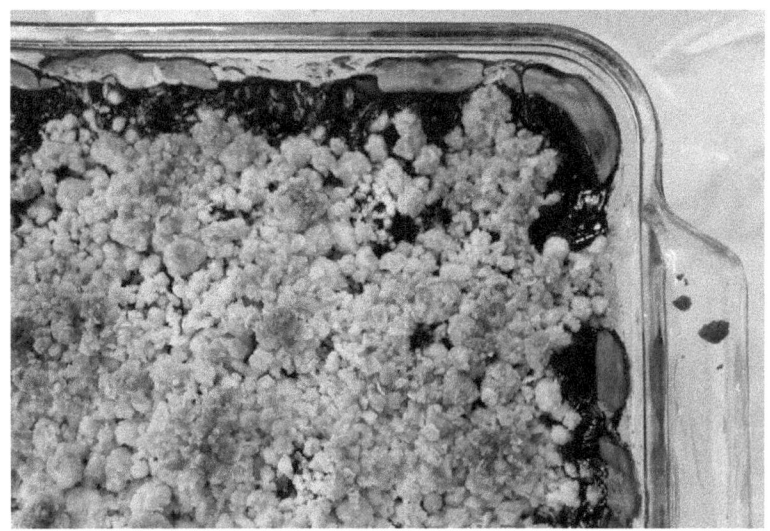

Chocolate Chip Quinoa Granola Bars

Preparation Time: 5 minutes

Cooking Time: 10 minutes

Servings: 16

Ingredients:

- ½ cup of chia seeds
- ½ cup walnuts, chopped
- 1 cup buckwheat
- 1 cup uncooked quinoa
- 2/3 cup dairy-free margarine
- ½ cup flax seed
- 1 teaspoon of cinnamon
- ½ cup of honey
- ½ cup of chocolate chips
- 1 teaspoon of vanilla
- ¼ teaspoon salt

Directions:

1. Preheat your oven to 350 degrees F.
2. Spread the walnuts, quinoa, wheat, flax, and chia on your baking sheet.
3. Bake for 10 minutes.

4. Line your baking dish with plastic wrap. Apply cooking spray. Keep aside.
5. Melt the margarine and honey in a saucepot.
6. Whisk together the vanilla, salt, and cinnamon into the margarine mix.
7. Keep the wheat mix and quinoa in a bowl. Pour the margarine sauce into it.
8. Stir the mixture. Coat well. Allow it to cool. Stir in the chocolate chips.
9. Spread your mixture into the baking dish. Press firmly into the pan.
10. Plastic wrap. Refrigerator overnight.
11. Slice into bars and serve.

Nutrition: Calories 408 Carbohydrates 31g Fat 28g Protein 8g Sugar 14g Fiber 6g Sodium 87mg

Strawberry Granita

Preparation Time: 10 minutes

Cooking Time: 10 minutes

Servings: 8

Ingredients:

- 2 lb. strawberries, halved & hulled
- 1 cup of water
- Agave to taste
- ¼ teaspoon balsamic vinegar
- ½ teaspoon lemon juice
- Just a small pinch of salt

Directions:

1. Rinse the strawberries in water.
2. Keep in a blender. Add water, agave, balsamic vinegar, salt, and lemon juice.
3. Pulse many times so that the mixture moves. Blend to make it smooth.
4. Pour into a baking dish. The puree should be 3/8 inch deep only.
5. Refrigerate the dish uncovered till the edges start to freeze. The center should be slushy.

6. Stir crystals from the edges lightly into the center. Mix thoroughly.
7. Chill till the granite is almost completely frozen.
8. Scrape loose the crystals like before and mix.
9. Refrigerate again. Use a fork to stir 3-4 times till the granite has become light.

Nutrition: Calories 72 Carbohydrates 17g FAT 0G Sugar 14g Fiber 2g Protein 1g

Apple Fritters

Preparation Time: 15 minutes

Cooking Time: 10 minutes

Servings: 4

Ingredients:
- 1 apple, cored, peeled, and chopped
- 1 cup all-purpose flour
- 1 egg
- ½ cup cashew milk
- 1-1/2 teaspoons of baking powder
- 2 tablespoons of stevia sugar

Directions:
1. Preheat your air fryer to 175 degrees C or 350 degrees F.
2. Keep parchment paper at the bottom of your fryer.
3. Apply cooking spray.
4. Mix together ¼ cup sugar, flour, baking powder, egg, milk, and salt in a bowl.
5. Combine well by stirring.
6. Sprinkle 2 tablespoons of sugar on the apples. Coat well.

7. Combine the apples into your flour mixture.
8. Use a cookie scoop and drop the fritters with it to the air fryer basket's bottom.
9. Now air fry for 5 minutes.
10. Flip the fritters once and fry for another 3 minutes. They should be golden.

Nutrition: Calories 307 Carbohydrates 65g Cholesterol 48mg Total Fat 3g Protein 5g Sugar 39g Fiber 2g Sodium 248mg

Roasted Bananas

Preparation Time: 2 minutes
Cooking Time: 7 minutes
Servings: 1
Ingredients:
- 1 banana, sliced into diagonal pieces
- Avocado oil cooking spray

Directions:
1. Take parchment paper and line the air fryer basket with it.
2. Preheat your air fryer to 190 degrees C or 375 degrees F.
3. Keep your slices of banana in the basket. They should not touch.
4. Apply avocado oil to mist the slices of banana.
5. Cook for 5 minutes.
6. Take out the basket. Flip the slices carefully.
7. Cook for 2 more minutes. The slices of banana should be caramelized and brown. Take them out from the basket.

Nutrition: Calories 121 Carbohydrates 27g Cholesterol 0mg Total Fat 1g Protein 1g Sugar 14g Fiber 3g

Sodium 1mg

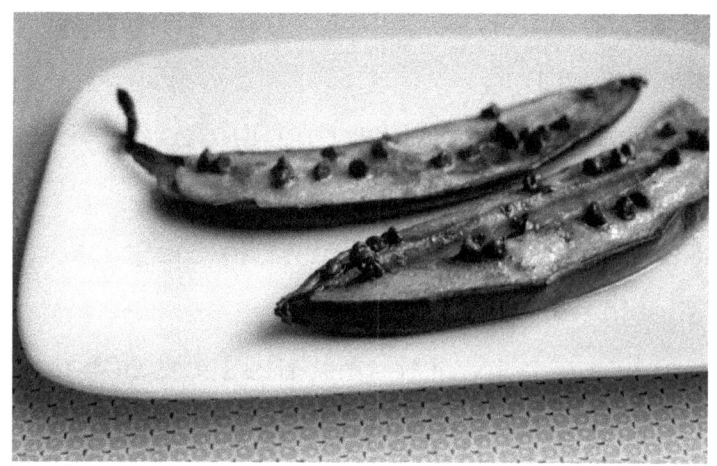

Berry-Banana Yogurt

Preparation Time: 10 minutes
Cooking Time: 0 minute
Servings: 1
Ingredients:

- ½ banana, frozen fresh
- 1 container 5.3ounes Greek yogurt, non-fat
- ¼ cup quick-cooking oats
- ½ cup blueberries, fresh and frozen
- 1 cup almond milk
- ¼ cup collard greens, chopped
- 5-6 ice cubes

Directions:

1. Take microwave-safe cup and add 1 cup almond milk and ¼ cup oats
2. Place the cups into your microwave on high for 2.5 minutes
3. When oats are cooked and 2 ice cubes to cool
4. Mix them well
5. Add all ingredients in your blender
6. Blend it until it gets a smooth and creamy mixture
7. Serve chilled and enjoy!

Nutrition: Calories: 379 Fat: 10g Carbohydrates: 63g Protein: 13g

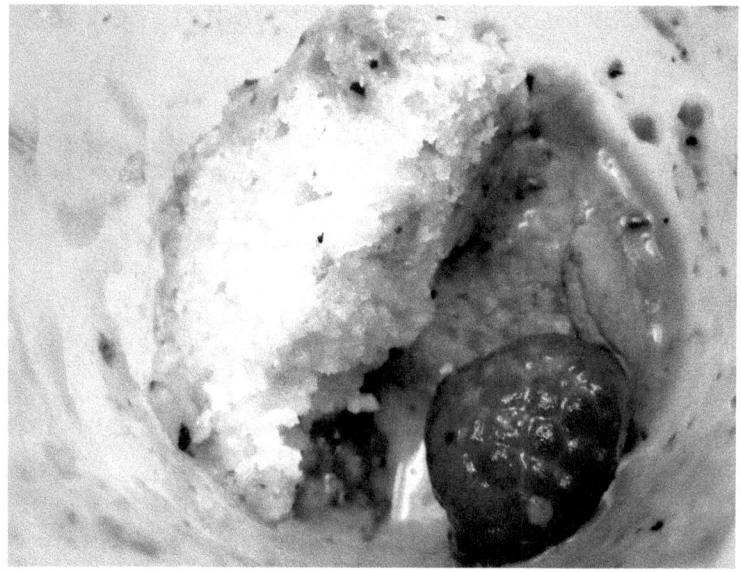

Avocado Chocolate Mousse

Preparation Time: 10 minutes

Cooking Time: 0 minute

Servings: 9

Ingredients:

- 3 ripe avocado, pitted and flesh scooped out
- 6 ounces plain Greek yogurt
- 1/8 cup almond milk, unsweetened
- ¼ cup espresso beans, ground
- ¼ cup of cocoa powder
- ½ teaspoon salt
- 2 tablespoons raw honey
- 1 bar dark chocolate
- 1 teaspoon vanilla extract

Directions:

1. Place all ingredients in your food processor
2. Pulse until smooth
3. Serve chilled and enjoy!

Nutrition: Calories: 208 Fat: 4g Carbohydrates: 17g Protein: 5g

Apricot Squares

Preparation Time: 20 minutes
Cooking Time: 0 minute
Servings: 8
Ingredients:

- 1 cup shredded coconut, dried
- 1 teaspoon vanilla extract
- 1 cup apricot, dried
- 1 cup macadamia nuts, chopped
- 1 cup apricot, chopped
- 1/3 cup turmeric powder

Directions:

1. Place all ingredients in your food processor
2. Pulse until smooth
3. Place the mixture into a square pan and press evenly
4. Serve chilled and enjoy!

Nutrition: Calories: 201 Fat: 15g Carbohydrates: 17g Protein: 3g

Raw Black Forest Brownies

Preparation Time: 2 hours and 10 minutes

Cooking Time: 0 minute

Servings: 6

Ingredients:

- 1 and ½ cups cherries, pitted, dried and chopped
- 1 cup raw cacao powder
- ½ cup dates pitted
- 2 cups walnuts, chopped
- ½ cup almonds, chopped
- ¼ teaspoon salt

Directions:

1. Place all ingredients in your food processor
2. Pulse until small crumbs are formed
3. Press the brownie batter in a pan
4. Freeze for two hours
5. Slice before serving and enjoy!

Nutrition: Calories: 294 Fat: 18g Carbohydrates: 33g Protein: 7g

Berry Parfait

Preparation Time: 10 min
Cooking Time: 10 min
Servings: 5
Ingredients:

- 7oz / 200g almond butter
- 3.5oz / 100g Greek yogurt
- 14oz / 400g mixed berries
- 2 tsp honey
- 7oz / 200g mixed nuts

Directions:

1. Mix the Greek yogurt, butter, and honey until it's smooth.
2. Add a layer of berries and a layer of the mixture in a glass until it's full.
3. Serve immediately with sprinkled nuts.

Nutrition: Calories: 250 Carbohydrates: 17 g Protein: 7.2 g Fat: 19.4 g Sugar: 42.3 g Fiber: 6.6 g Sodium: 21 mg

Sherbet Pineapple

Preparation Time: 20 Minutes
Cooking Time: 0 Minute
Servings: 4
Ingredients:
- 1 can of 8-ounce pineapple chunks
- 1/3 cup of orange marmalade
- ¼ teaspoon of ground ginger
- ¼ teaspoon of vanilla extract
- 1 can of 11-ounce orange sections
- 2 cups of pineapple, lemon or lime sherbet

Directions:
1. Drain the pineapple, ensure you reserve the juice.
2. Take a medium-sized bowl and add pineapple juice, ginger, vanilla and marmalade to the bowl
3. Add pineapple chunks, drained mandarin oranges as well
4. Toss well and coat everything
5. Free them for 15 minutes and allow them to chill
6. Spoon the sherbet into 4 chilled stemmed sherbet dishes

7. Top each of them with fruit mixture
8. Enjoy!

Nutrition: Calories: 267 Cal Fat: 1 gCarbohydrates: 65 g Protein: 2 g

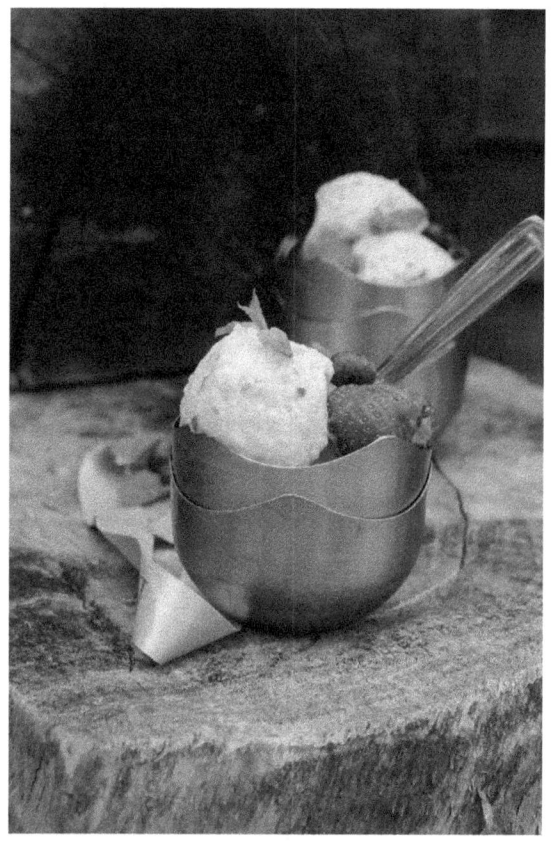

SNACKS

Blueberry Scones

Preparation Time: 5 minutes
Cooking Time: 25 minutes
Servings: 2
Ingredients:

- 2 cups almond flour
- 1/3 cup Swerve sweetener
- ¼ cup coconut flour
- 1 tbsp. baking powder
- ¼ tsp salt
- 2 large eggs
- ¼ cup heavy whipping cream
- ½ tsp vanilla extract
- ¾ cup fresh blueberries

Directions:

1. Preheat your oven at 325 degrees F. Layer a baking sheet with wax paper.
2. Whisk almond flour with baking powder, salt, coconut flour, and sweetener in a large bowl.

3. Stir in eggs, vanilla, and cream then mix well until fully incorporated.
4. Add blueberries and mix gently.
5. Spread this dough on a baking sheet and form it into a 10x8-inch rectangle.
6. Bake these scones for 25 minutes until golden.
7. Allow them to cool then serve.

Nutrition: Calories: 266 Fat 25.7 g Saturated Fat 1.2 g Cholesterol 41 Sodium 18

Homemade Graham Crackers

Preparation Time: 5 minutes
Cooking Time: 30 minutes
Servings: 12
Ingredients:

- 2 cups almond flour
- 1/3 cup Swerve Brown
- 2 tsp cinnamon
- 1 tsp baking powder
- Pinch salt
- 1 large egg
- 2 tbsp. butter, melted
- 1 tsp vanilla extract

Directions:

1. Preheat your oven at 300 degrees F.
2. Whisk almond flour, baking powder, salt, cinnamon, and sweetener in a large bowl.
3. Stir in melted butter, egg, and vanilla extract.
4. Mix well to form the dough then spread it out into a ¼-inch thick sheet.
5. Slice the sheet into 2x2-inch squares and place them on a baking sheet with wax paper.
6. Bake them for 30 minutes until golden then let them sit for 30 minutes at room temperature until cooled.

7. Break the crackers into smaller squares and put them back in the hot oven for 30 minutes. Keep the oven off during this time.
8. Enjoy.

Nutrition: Calories: 243 Fat: 21 g Cholesterol: 121 Sodium: 34 Carb0hydrates: 7.3 Protein: 4.3 g

Lightning Source UK Ltd.
Milton Keynes UK
UKHW051100150121
377077UK00016B/277